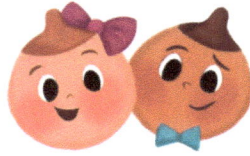

For Lea, Jordan & Michael
& anyone who has ever felt
uncomfortable with their boobs
(myself included!)

EVERYONE Has BOOBiES!

Written by
Dr. Robyn Roth

Illustrated by
Amna

Last week in class, our teacher said,
"We have a **special** guest!"

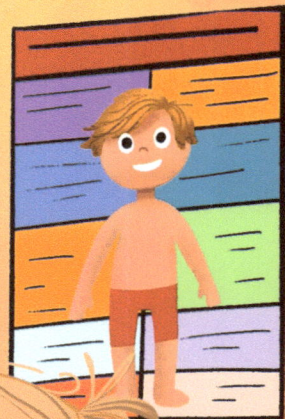
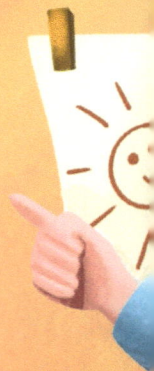
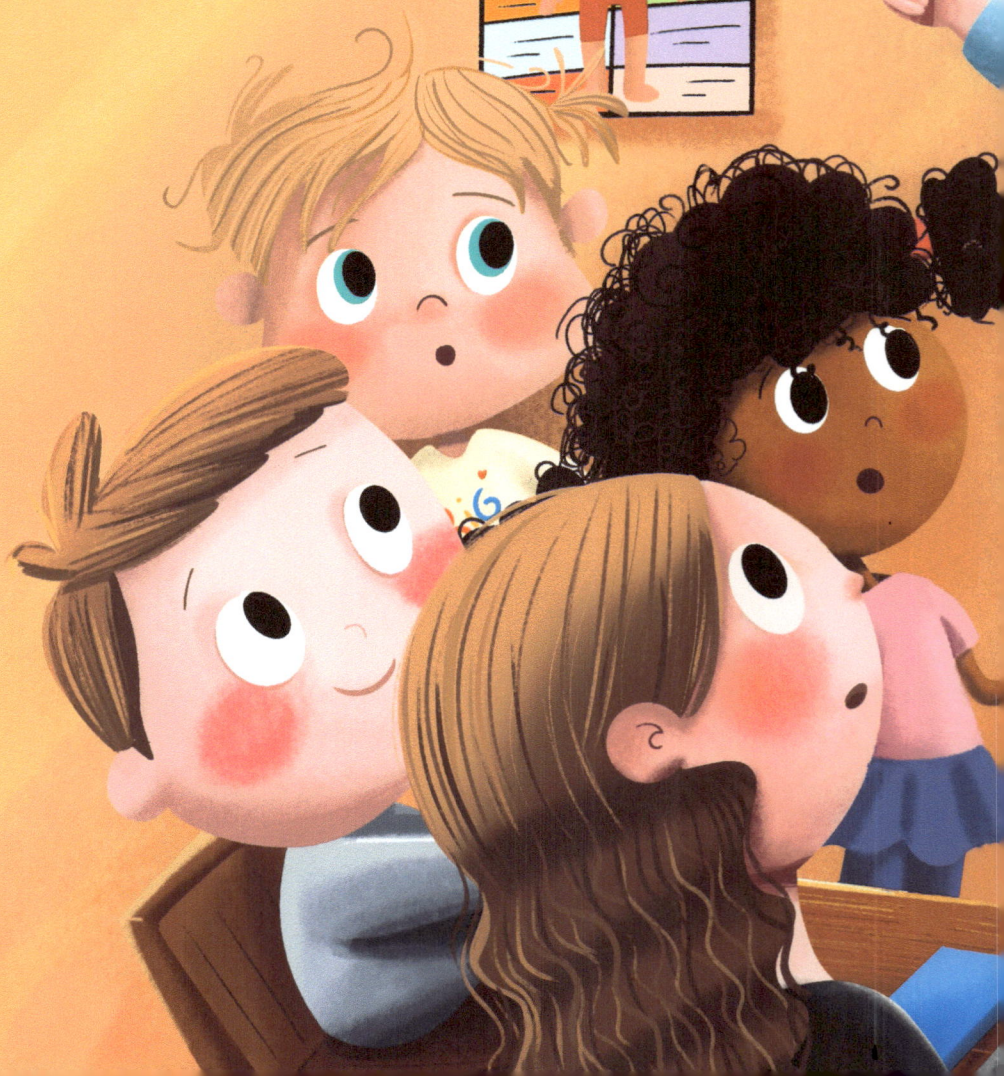

2+2=4

The door swung wide,
and to our surprise, who walked in?
A breast!

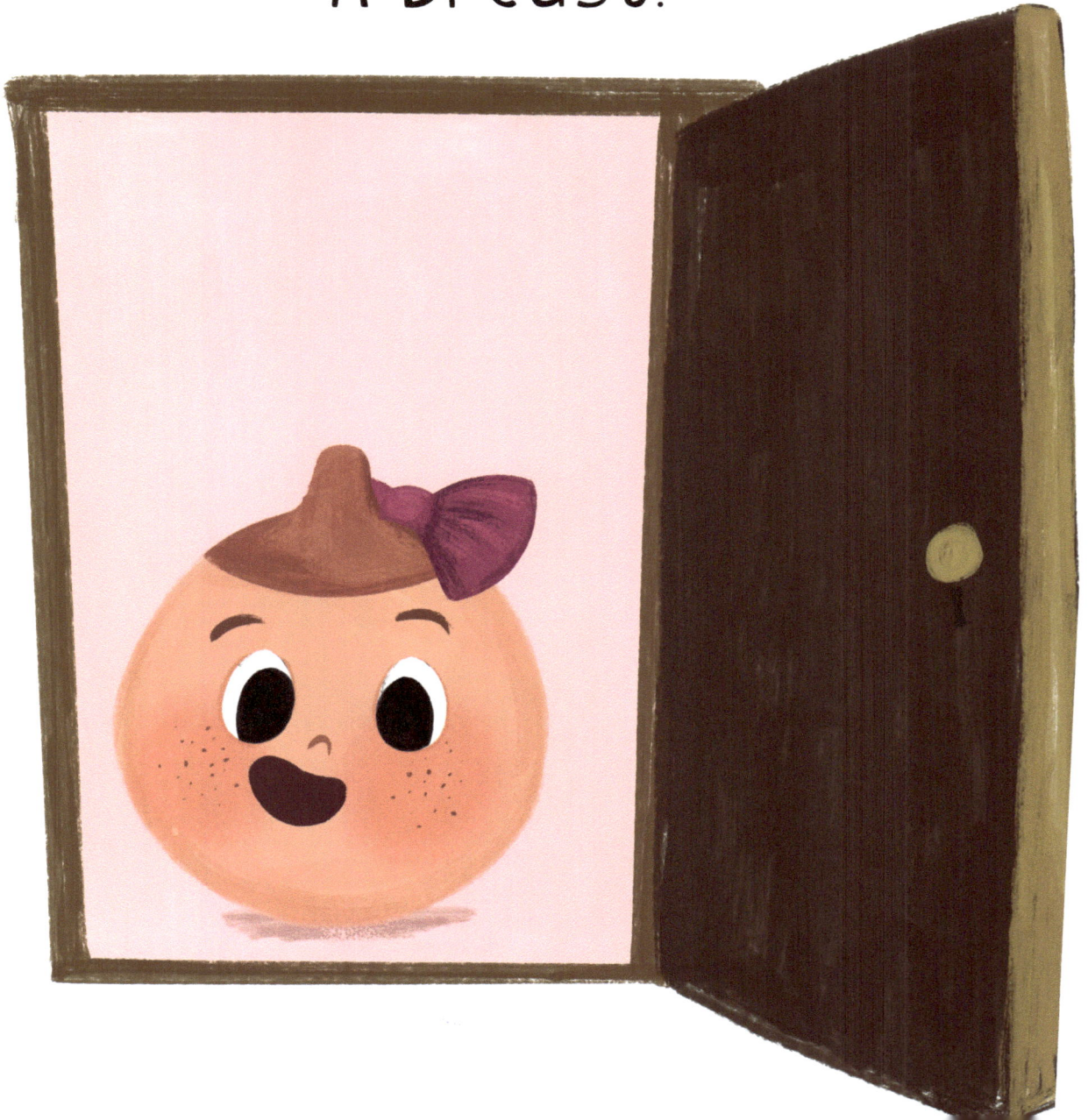

The class began to chuckle,
followed with blank stares.
"Hey kids, I'm just a boobie!
There's no reason to be scared."

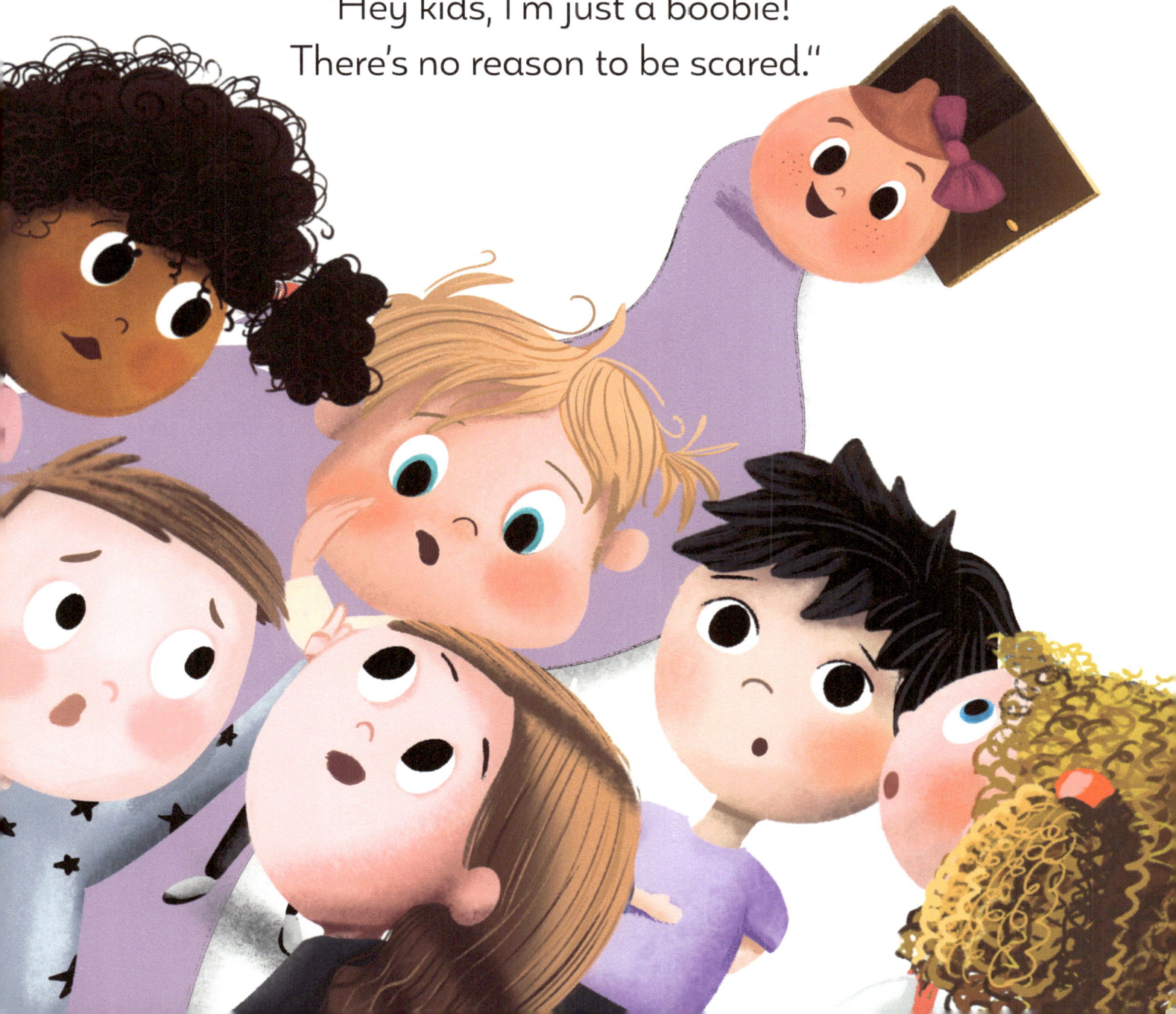

"Everyone has boobies, it's pretty plain to see.
Everyone has boobies,

just like YOU and me."

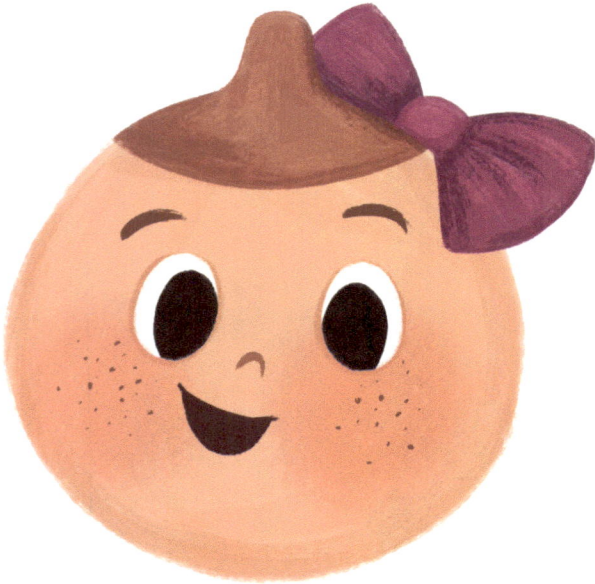
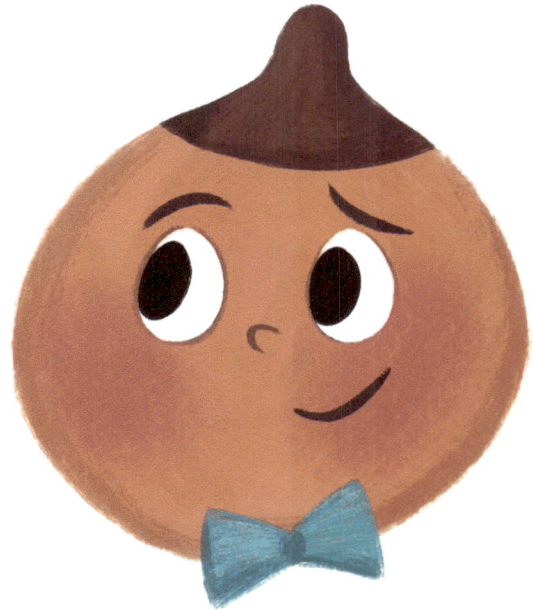

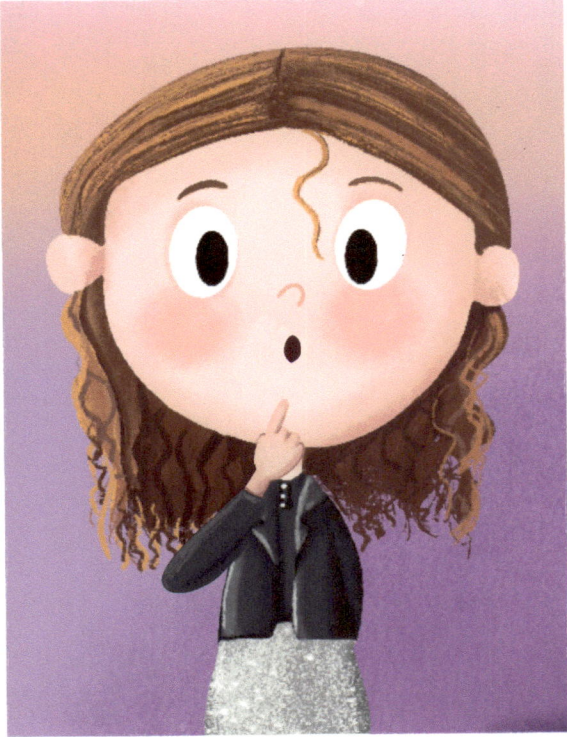

"Hey! You can't say those words, the ones that start with B!"

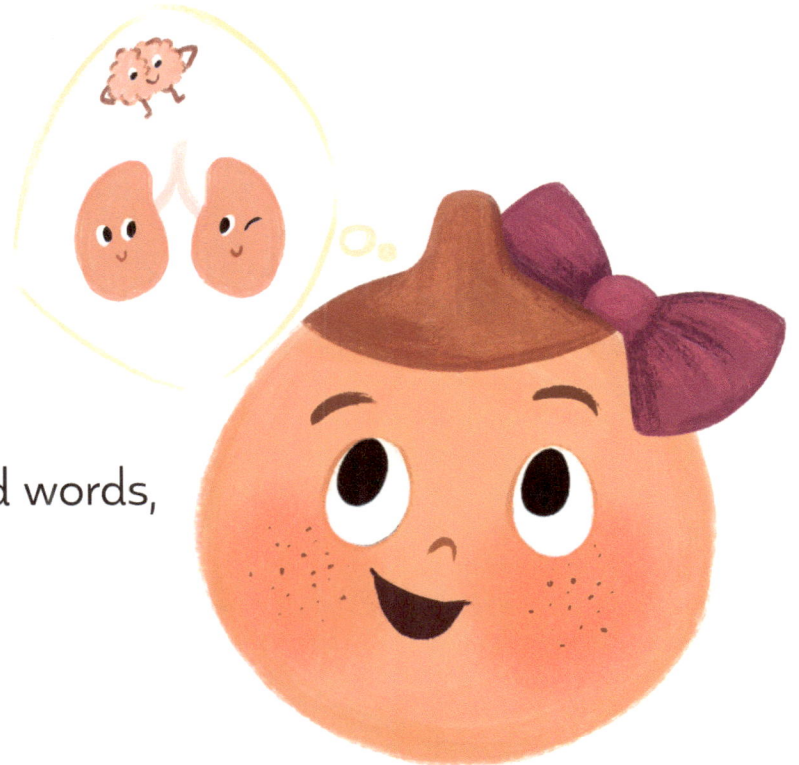

"Breasts & boobies aren't bad words, it's just anatomy."

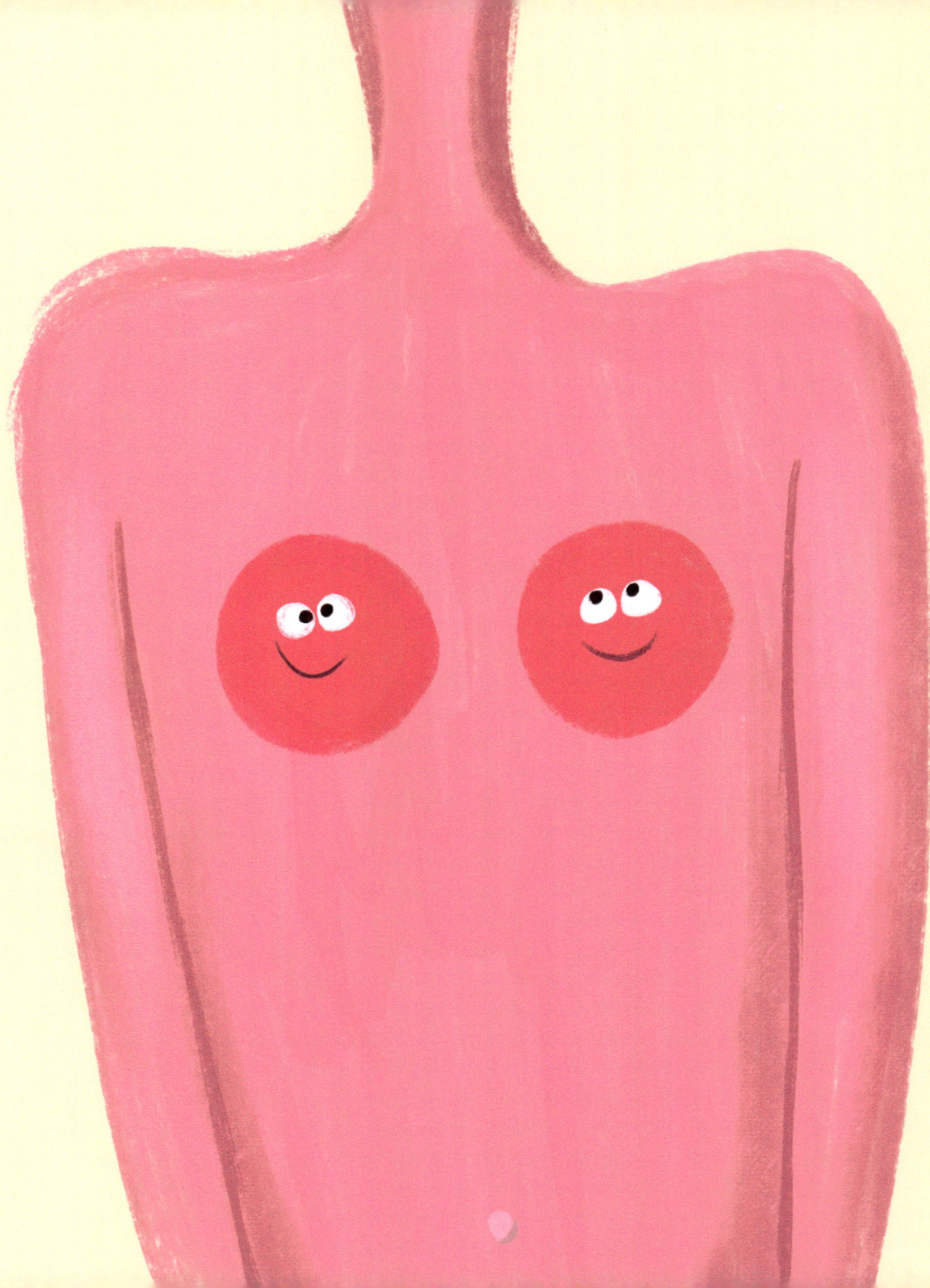

Boobs

Boobies

Breasts

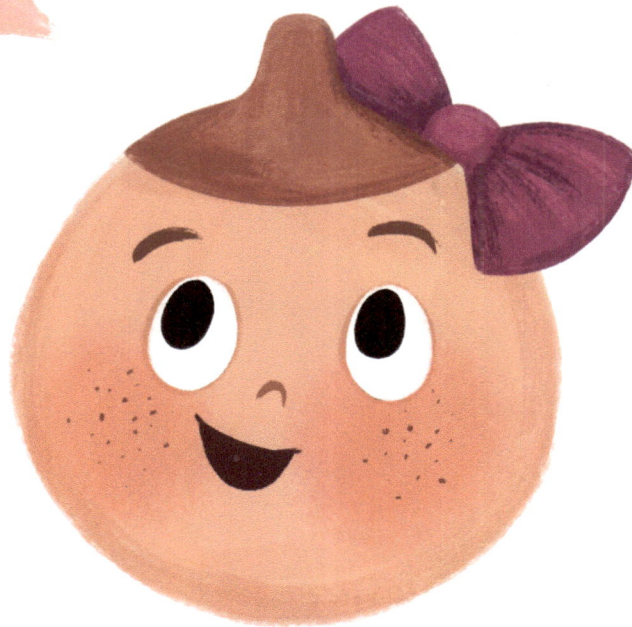

"You can call them what you like—
boobs, boobies, breasts.
They're blobs of glands, fat, and tissue
just sitting on your chest."

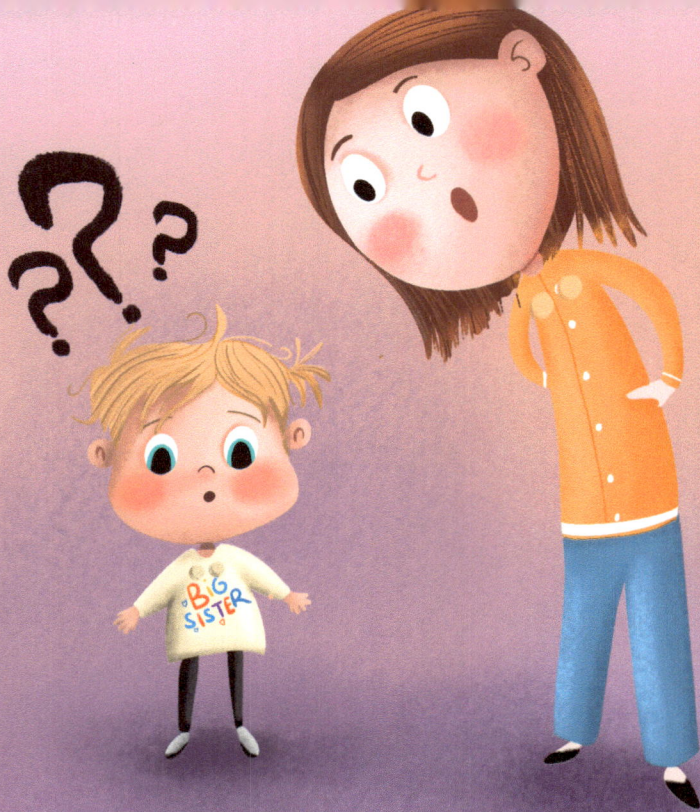

"Our boobies grow as we grow,
some are **big** and some are little.
Did you know boys have boobies too?
You have permission to **giggle**!"

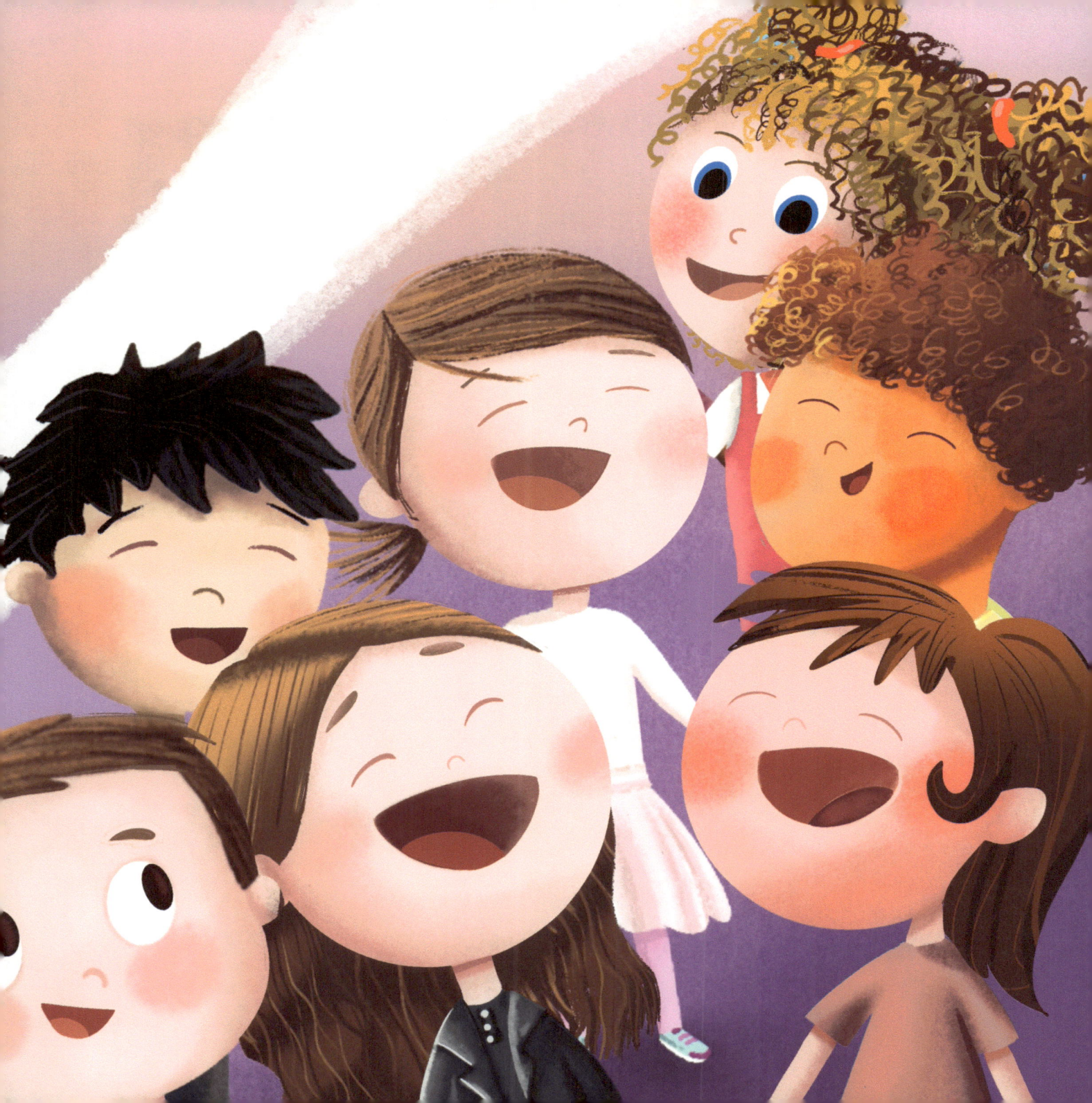

"And while we sit & giggle,
let's talk about the **nipple**!
Most people have two but not all do,
so it's really not that simple."

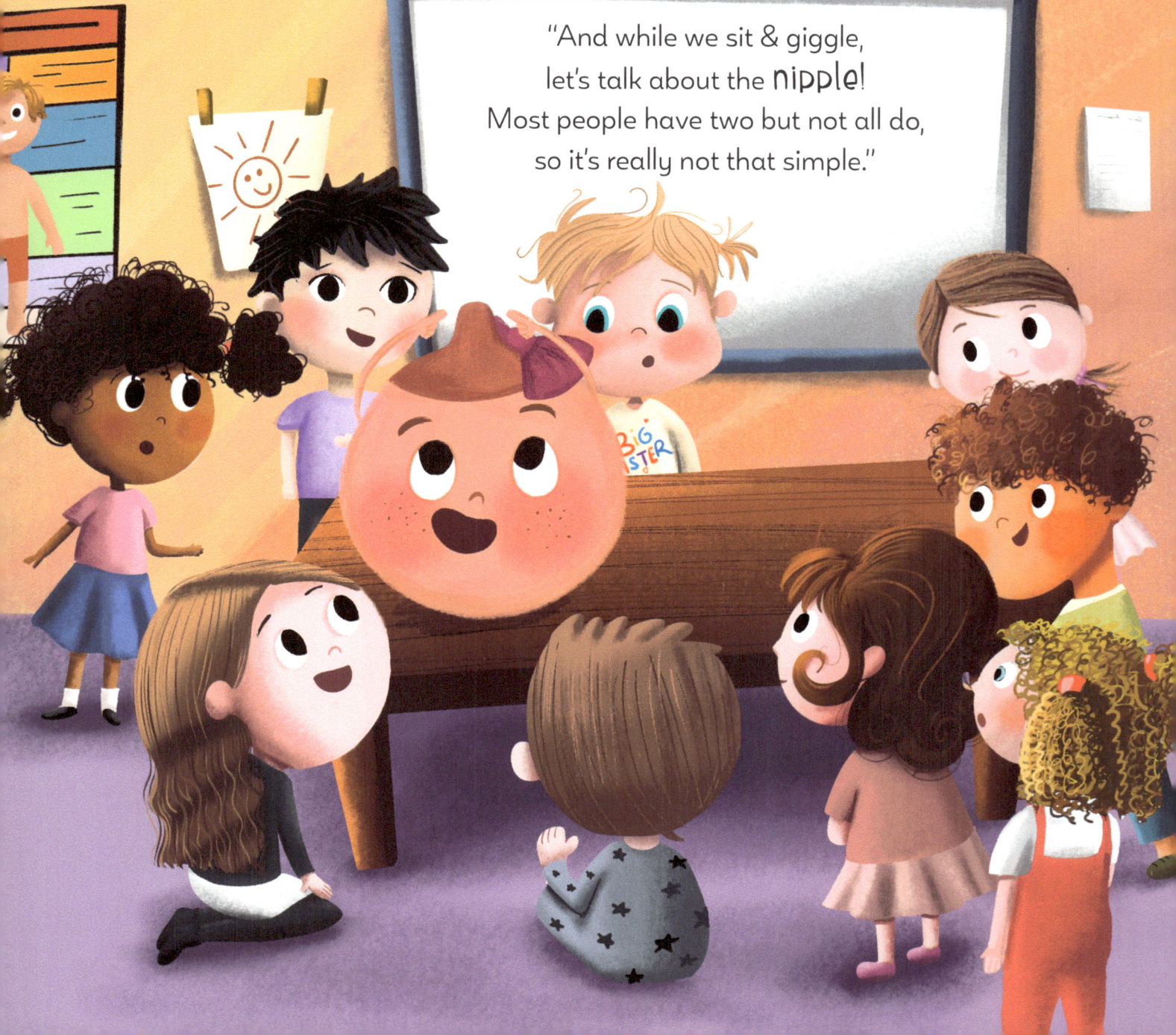

"Mommy's boobies can make milk
to feed babies when they're small.
They offer food & comfort!"

"Wow,
boobies do it all!"

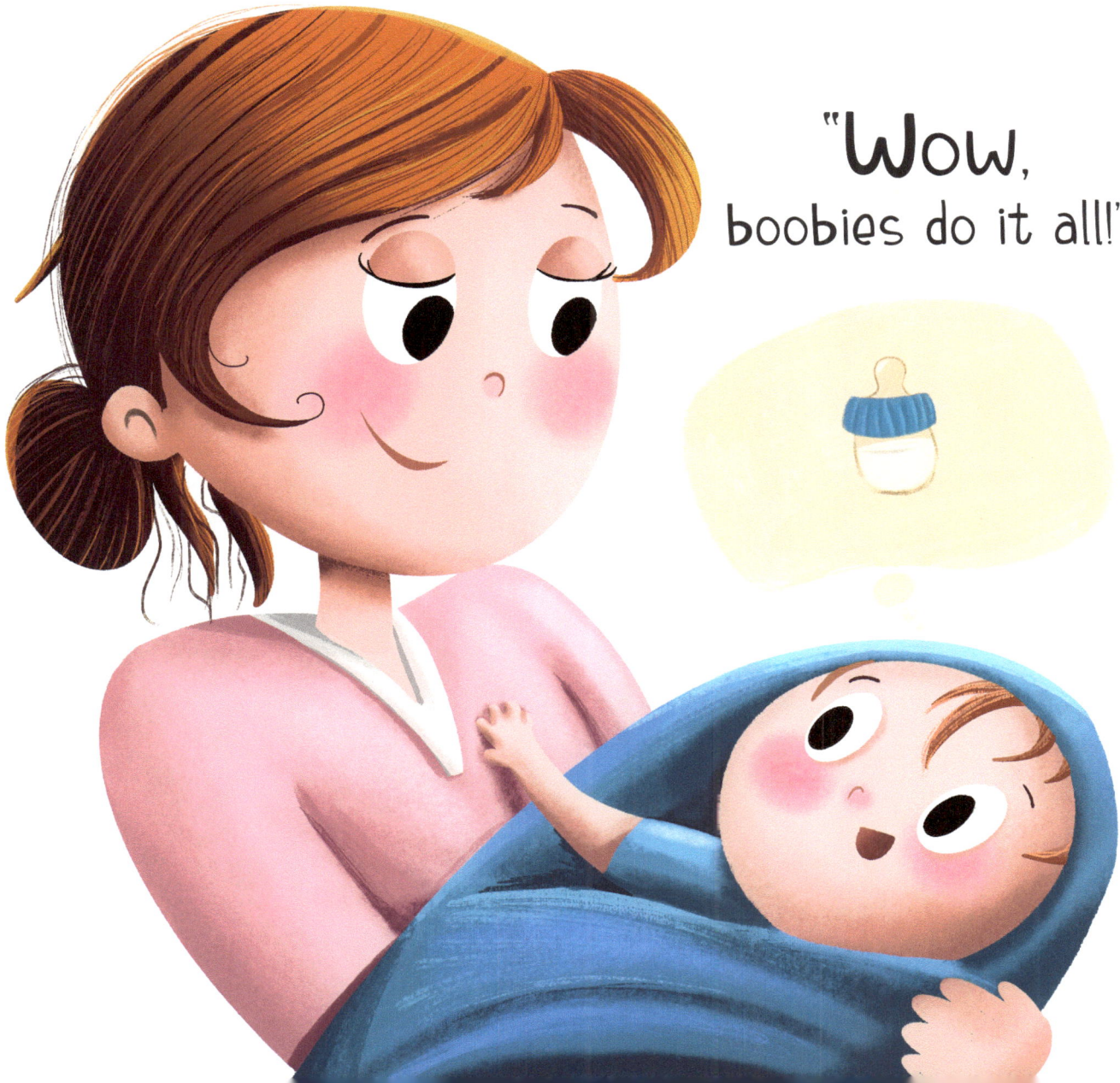

"Do animals have **boobies?**"
"Yes, all mammals do!
Mice have 10, pigs have 12.
Goats and elephants have 2."

Mice have 10

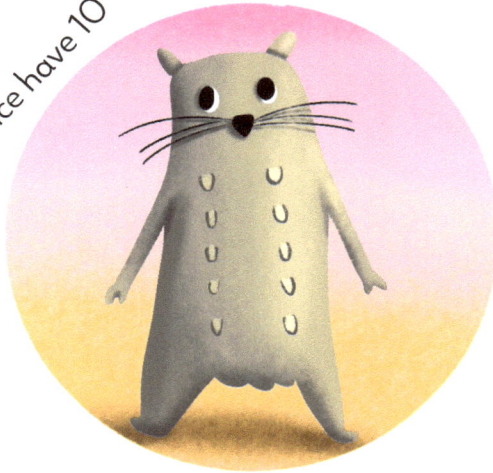

Pigs have 12

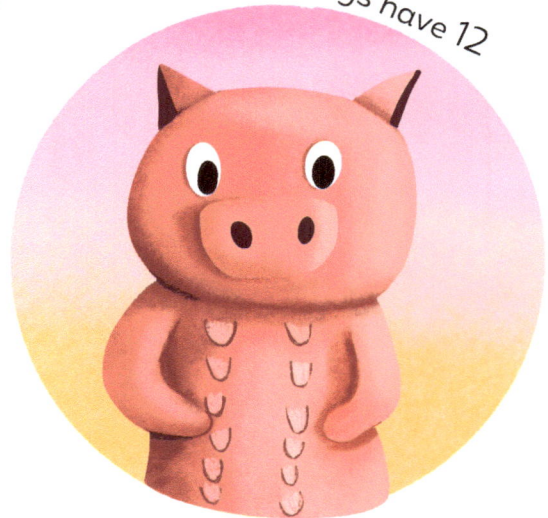

Goats have 2

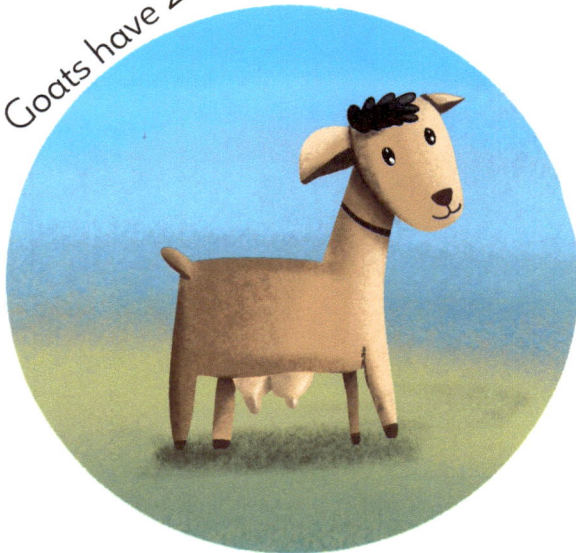

"Cows have 4, and some have more,
like bears and cats and rats."

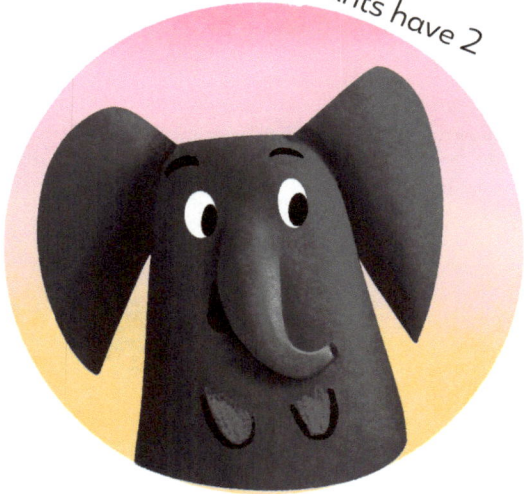

Elephants have 2

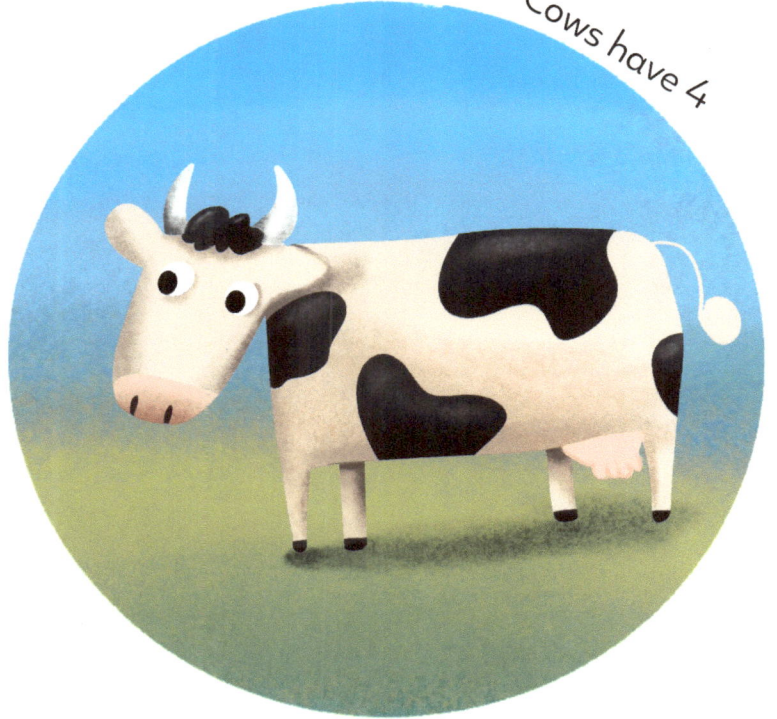

Cows have 4

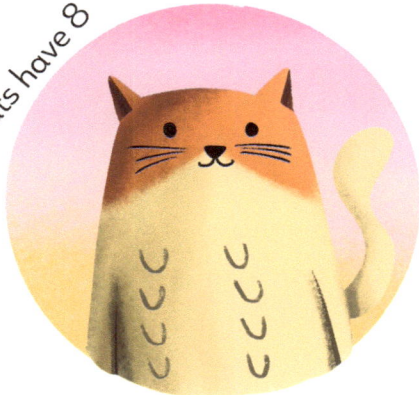

Cats have 8

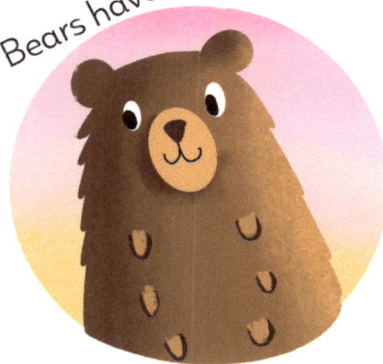

Bears have 6

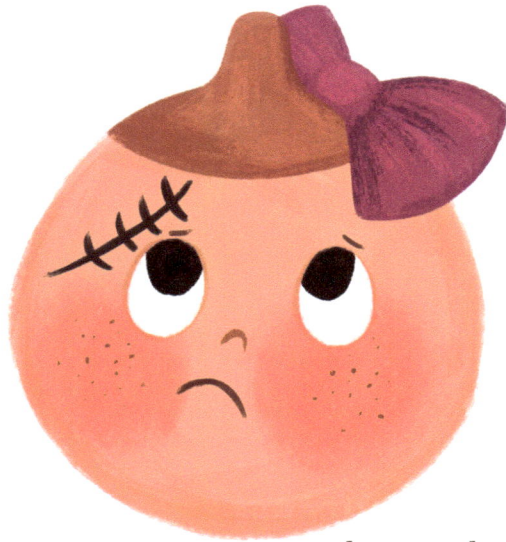

"But boobies can get **boo-boos**,
and have a scar or two."

"My mommy's boobies have a scar."
"My daddy has one too."

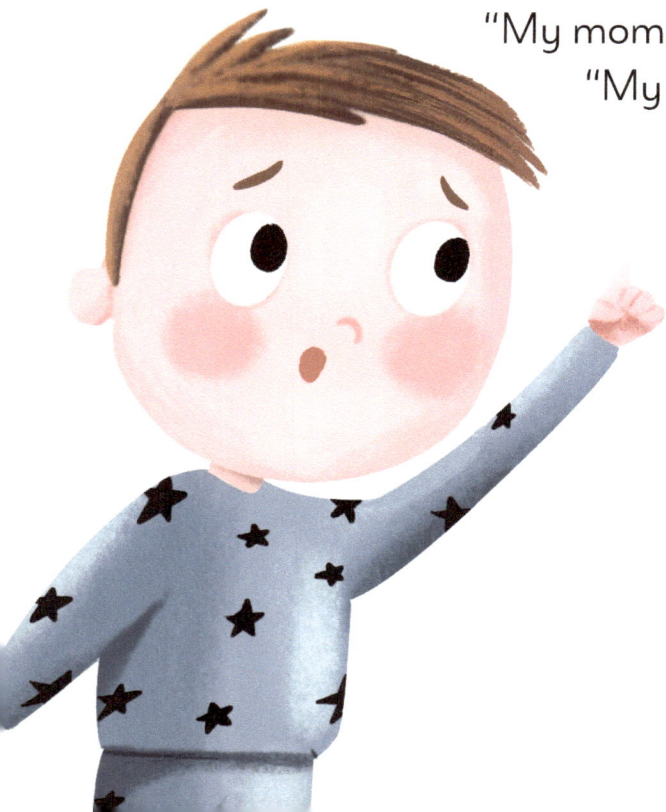

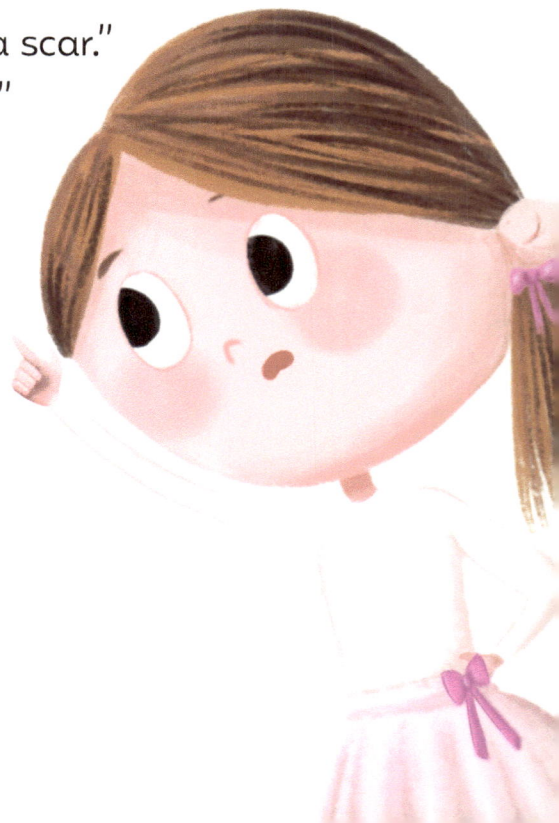

"But if boobies get a **boo-boo**,
there are things that doctors can do!
They can **find** it, they can **shrink** it,
They can **fry** it , they can **freeze** it,
they can **cut** it, they can **cure** it,
& make that boobie boo-boo **go**
bye bye bye!"

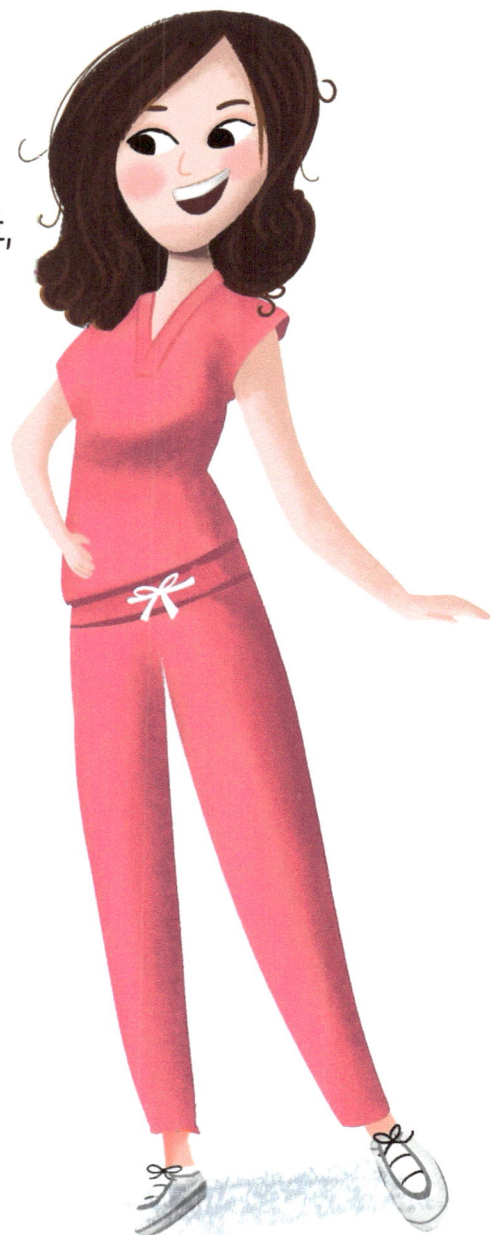

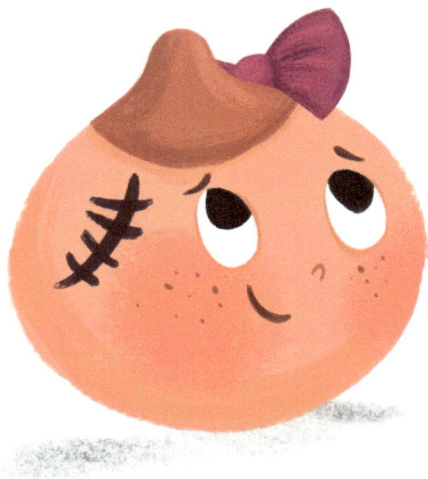

"Boobies come in all **shapes** and **sizes**,
no two are the same!
Boobies are special just like us,
no need to be ashamed!"

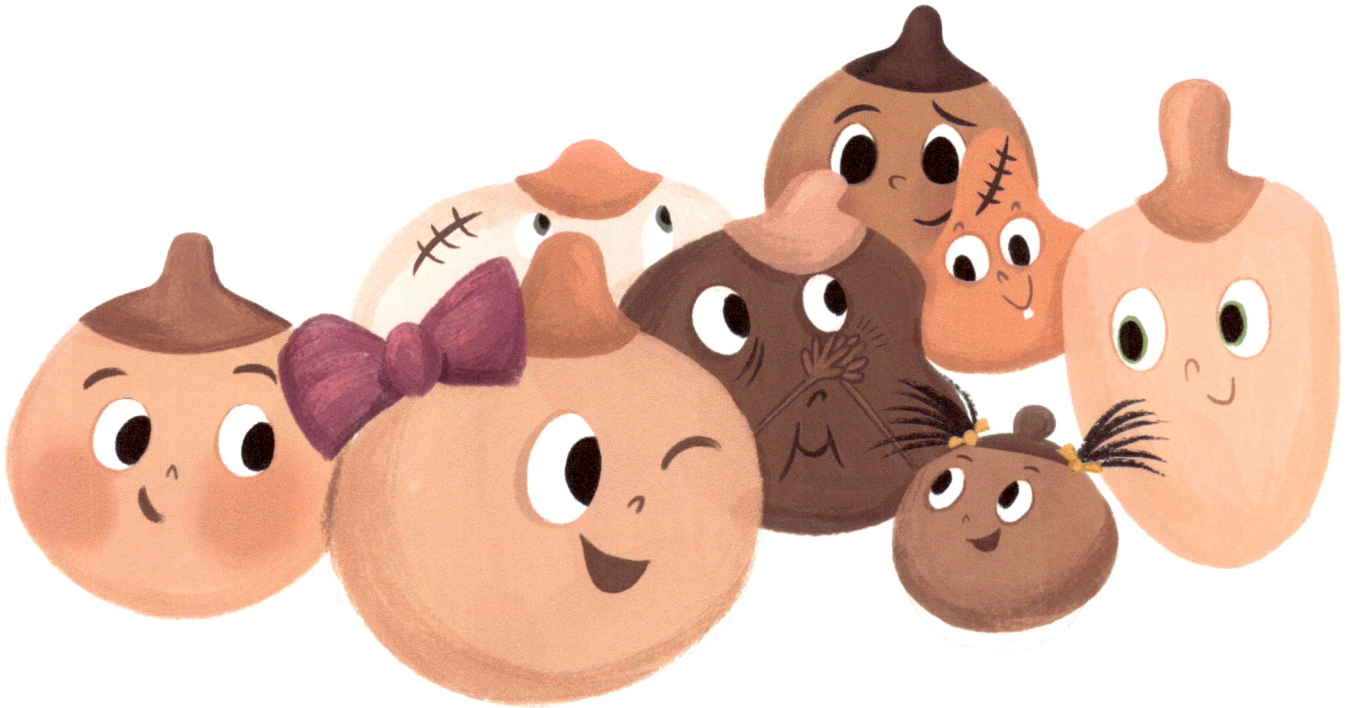

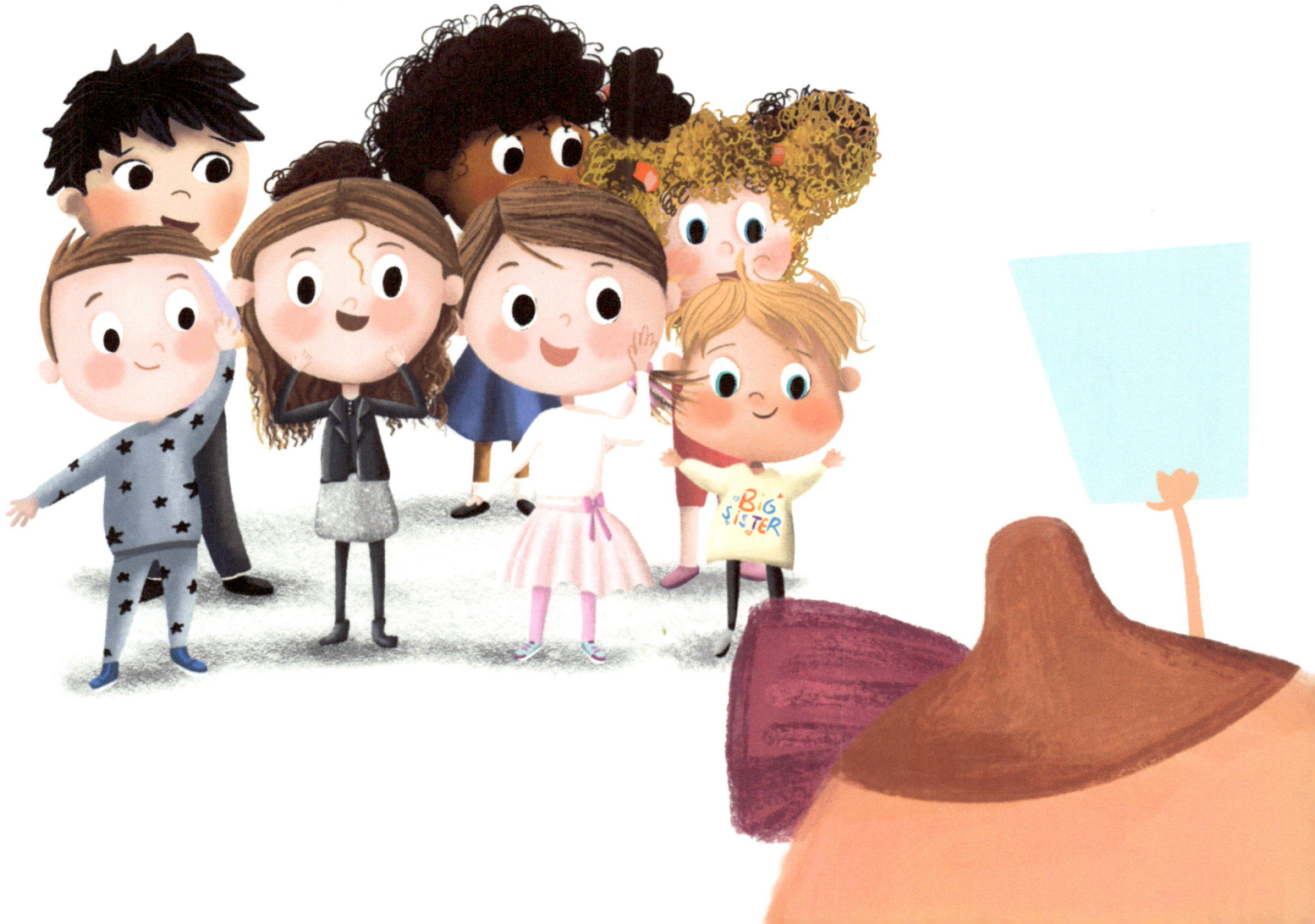

"So don't be scared of boobies,
they're parts of our bodies!

Now let's count together, 1.2.3,
and say boobies after me!"

1...... 2.......... 2 ½ .... 3!

BOOBIES!
Now like a ghost... Booooooo-bies!

RO-BOT BOO-BIES!
PEEKA-BOOB!

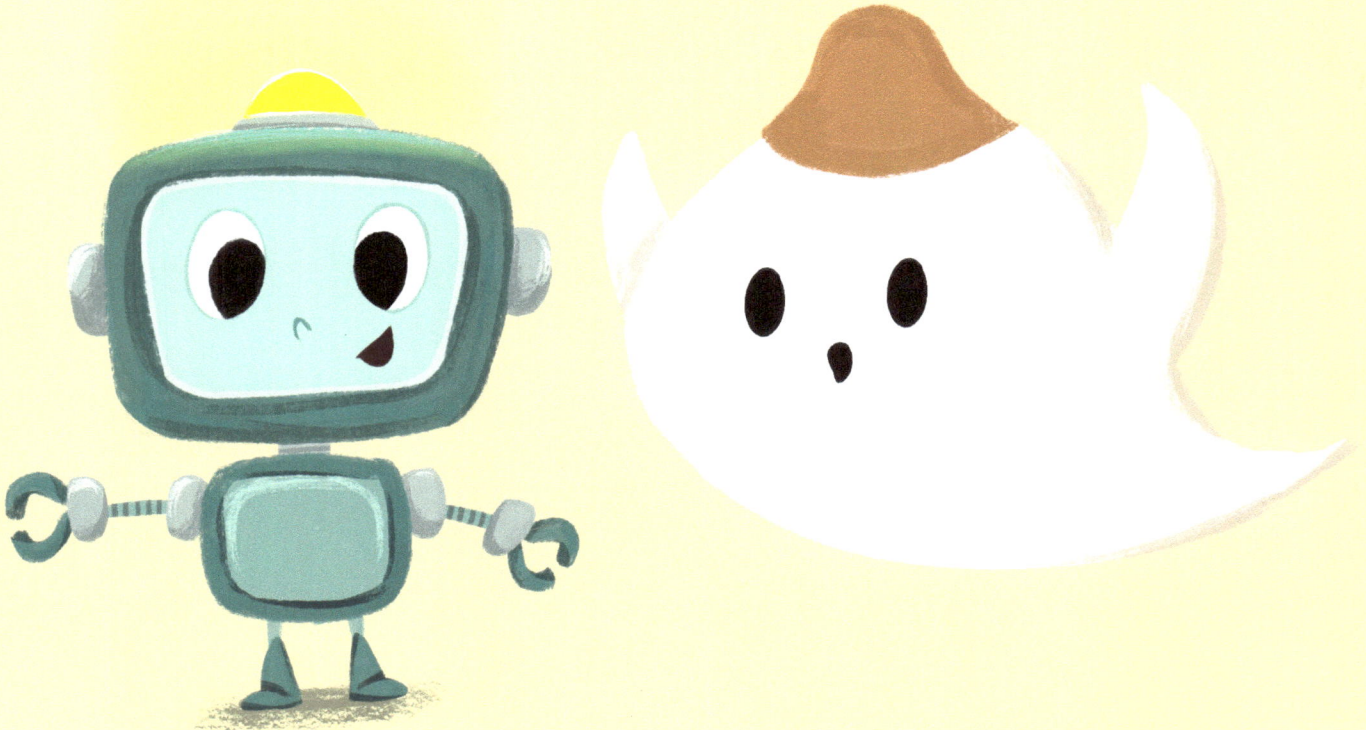

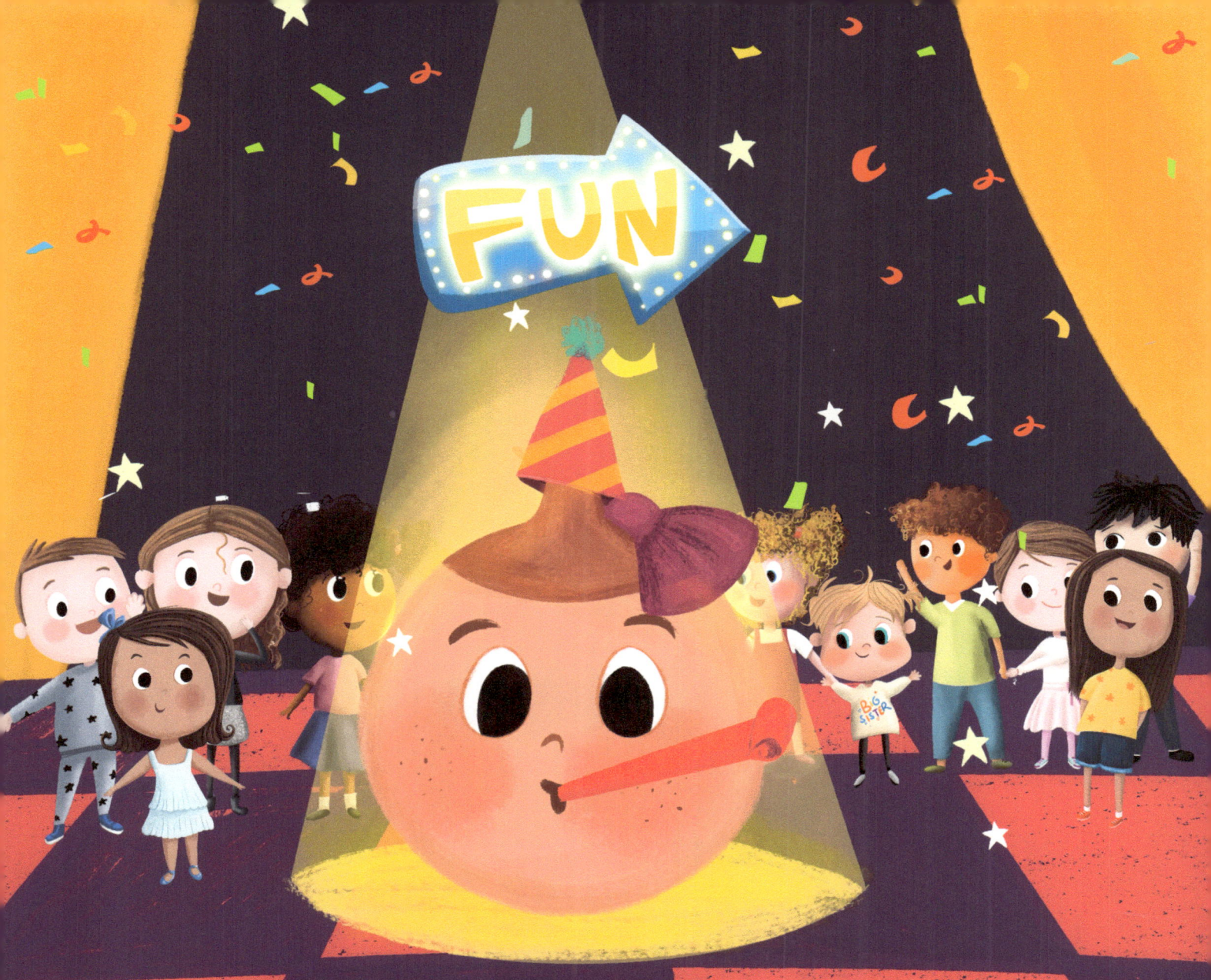

See, isn't learning about breasts FUN?!

"So take care of your boobies,
and treat them with respect.
They deserve your love, from up above

because boobies are the best!"

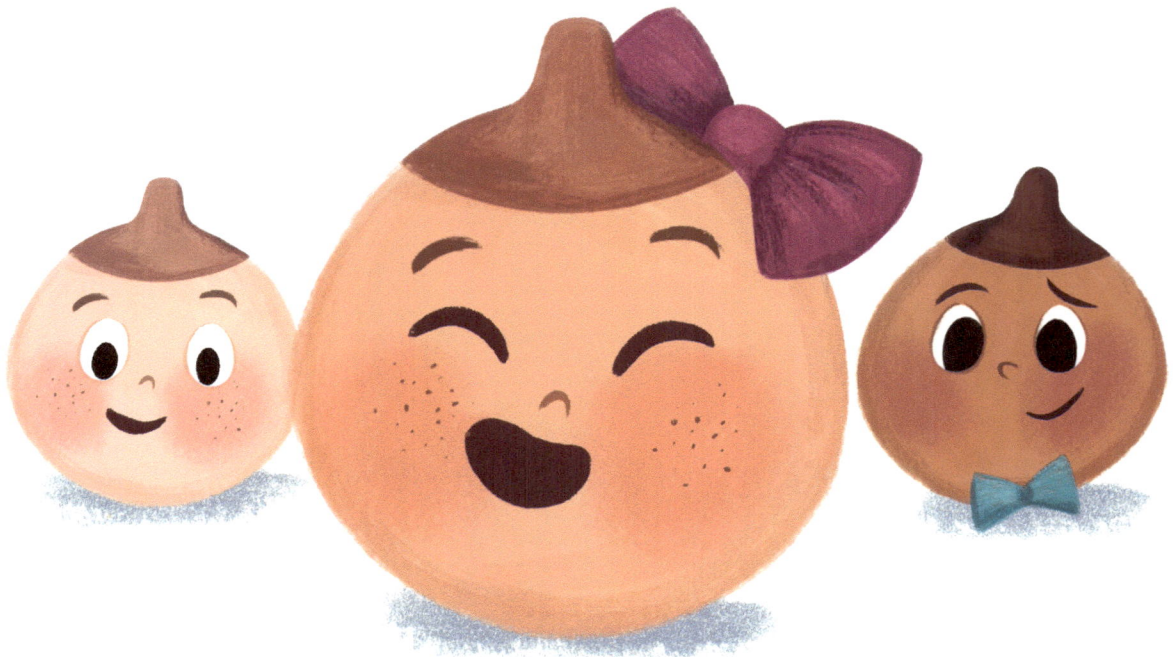

Meet the Author

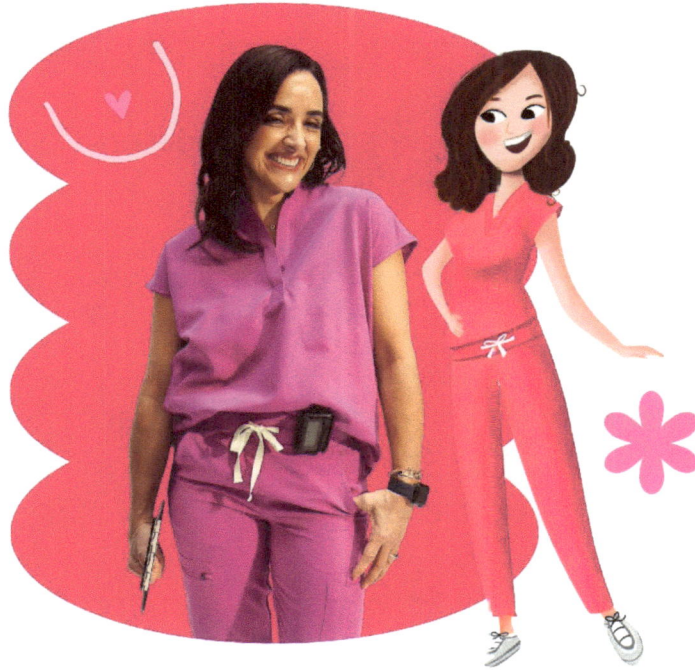

Dr. Robyn Roth is a board-certified breast radiologist.
Her friends call her **@TheBoobieDocs,** her popular
social media platform where she discusses
breast health in an educational and fun way.
She lives in Southern New Jersey with her husband and
3 young children. She has 2 breasts.

Learn more at **theboobiedocs.com!**

If your boobie has a boo-boo, here are resources that can help you.

Bright Spot Network- Virtual support groups for parents or caregivers going through cancer while raising young children

Pickles Group- Peer-to-peer support and resources for kids and teens impacted by their parent's cancer.

Sharsheret- Help guide your children through your cancer or prophylactic surgery journey with the Sharsheret Busy Box which contains resources and activities to occupy your children while you are at the doctor or resting after treatment.

Wonders & Worries- Provides free, professional support for children and teenagers through a parent's serious illness or injury.

Camp Kesem- Free summer camps and year-round support for children whose parents have or had cancer. Helps kids connect with peers.

Family Reach- Financial support and help with basics for families facing cancer.

American Cancer Society (ACS)- Helpline, navigation support, resources for families and caregivers, help managing insurance and finances.

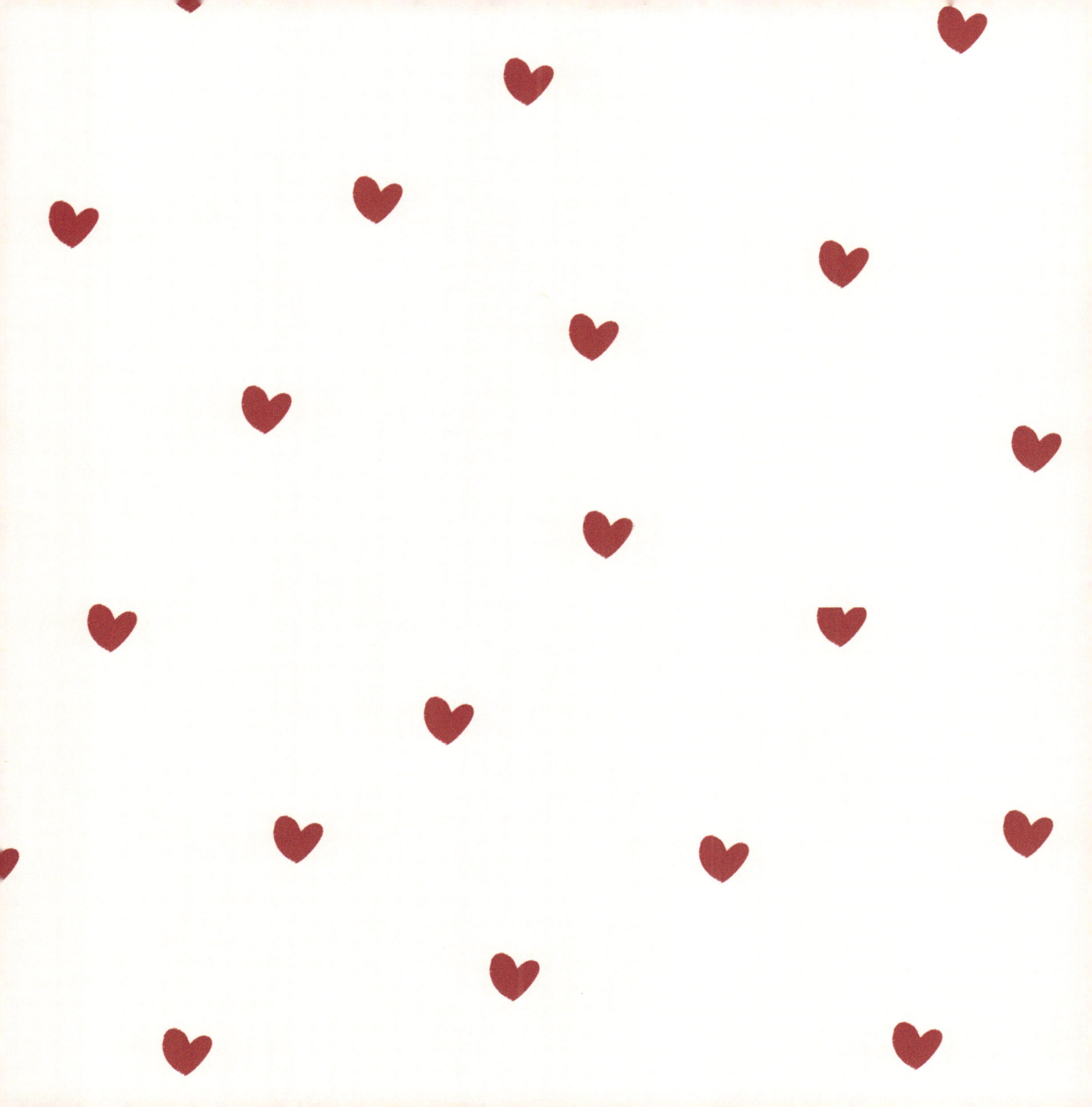

www.ingramcontent.com/pod-product-compliance
Lightning Source LLC
Chambersburg PA
CBHW060828270326
41931CB00002B/99